PHARMACEUTICS-I

(PRACTICAL NOTEBOOK)
FOR
1st YEAR DIPLOMA IN PHARMACY

(According to the new syllabus as prescribed by Pharmacy Council of India, Education Regulation 1991, implemented in the year 1993, for Pharmaceutics-I students)

By
A. GUPTA
and
V.K. JAIN

Name of Student	. . . .
Roll No.	. . . .
College	. . . .
	. . . .

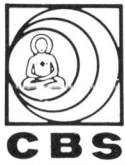

CBS

CBS Publishers & Distributors Pvt. Ltd.
New Delhi • Bengaluru • Chennai • Kochi • Kolkata • Mumbai
Hyderabad • Nagpur • Patna • Pune • Vijayawada

ISBN: 81-239-0683-8

First Edition: 1996
Reprint: 1998, 1999, 2000, 2003, 2004, 2005, 2006, 2007, 2008
      2010, 2011, 2012, 2014, 2015, 2016, 2018, 2019, 2020, 2021

Published by **Satish Kumar Jain** and produced by **Varun Jain** for
CBS Publishers & Distributors Pvt. Ltd.,
4819/XI Prahlad Street, 24 Ansari Road, Daryaganj, New Delhi - 110002
delhi@cbspd.com, cbspubs@airtelmail.in • www.cbspd.com
Ph.: 23289259, 23266861, 23266867 • Fax: 011-23243014

Corporate Office: 204 FIE, Industrial Area, Patparganj, Delhi - 110 092
Ph: 49344934 • Fax: 011-49344935
E-mail: publishing@cbspd.com • publicity@cbspd.com

Branches:
- *Bengaluru:* 2975, 17th Cross, K.R. Road, Bansankari 2nd Stage,
  Bengaluru - 70 • Ph: +91-80-26771678/79 • Fax: +91-80-26771680
  E-mail: cbsbng@gmail.com, bangalore@cbspd.com
- *Chennai:* No. 7, Subbaraya Street, Shenoy Nagar, Chennai - 600030
  Ph: +91-44-26681266, 26680620 • Fax: +91-44-42032115
  E-mail: chennai@cbspd.com
- *Kochi:* Ashana House, 39/1904, A.M. Thomas Road, Valanjambalam,
  Ernakulum, Kochi • Ph: +91-484-4059061-65
  Fax: +91-484-4059065 • E-mail: cochin@cbspd.com
- *Kolkata:* 6-B, Ground Floor, Rameshwar Shaw Road, Kolkata - 700014
  Ph: +91-33-22891126/7/8 • E-mail: kolkata@cbspd.com
- *Mumbai:* 83-C, Dr. E. Moses Road, Worli, Mumbai - 400018
  Ph: +91-9833017933, 022-24902340/41 • E-mail: mumbai@cbspd.com

Representatives:

• Hyderabad: 0-9885175004	• Nagpur: 0-9021734563
• Patna: 0-9334159340	• Pune: 0-9623451994
• Jharkhand: 0-9811541605	• Uttarakhand: 0-9716462459

Printed at: India Binding House, Noida, UP

Preface

According to Education Regulation 1991 of the Pharmacy Council of India, implemented in the year 1993, students of Diploma in Pharmacy, 1st year are required to prepare at least 30 preparations in Pharmaceutics-I subject. This Practical Manual has been written keeping in view the new syllabus as prescribed by P.C.I. and also the difficulties faced by students and teachers.

This Practical Manual contains 31 exercises and they cover all the topics mentioned in the syllabus. The topics covered are Aromatic Waters, Solutions, Spirits, Tinctures, Extracts, Creams, Cosmetic Preparations, Capsules, Tablets, Preparations Involving Sterilisation (Parenteral Preparations), Ophthalmic Preparations, Preparations Involving Aseptic Techniques.

The preparations have been discussed in a very simple language and in detail. At the end of this Practical Manual, a few pages have been left blank for notes to be made by students. Left-hand side page facing every exercise has been left blank. The students can write calculations, method of preparation in their own language, etc., on these pages.

AUTHORS

Syllabus (Pharmaceutics-I)

As per Pharmacy Council of India, time allotted for Pharmaceutics-I practicals is 100 hours. Given below is the list of topics and number of exercises in each topic.

Topics	Number of Exercises
1. Aromatic Waters	3
2. Solutions	4
3. Spirits	2
4. Tinctures	4
5. Extracts	2
6. Creams	2
7. Cosmetic Preparations	3
8. Capsules	2
9. Tablets	2
10. Preparations Involving Sterilisation	2
11. Ophthalmic Preparations	2
12. Preparations Involving Aseptic Techniques	2

Contents

INDEX

S. No.	Name of Exercise	Date	Page	Remarks

INDEX

S. No.	Name of Exercise	Date	Page	Remarks

1

Aromatic Waters

Aromatic waters, also known as medicated waters, are clear saturated solutions of volatile oils or other aromatic or volatile substances in water. Their odours and tastes are similar to those of volatile oils or volatile substances from which they are prepared. The volatile substances from which the aromatic waters are to be prepared should be of highest quality.

Aromatic waters are mainly used for their flavouring properties as vehicles for the internal administration of medicaments or they are used as menstruum for the extraction of drugs due to their flavouring, sweetening and preservative properties. Some of the aromatic waters have a mild therapeutic action due to their carminative properties.

There are two types of aromatic waters which are described below :

(a) Simple aromatic waters

Simple aromatic waters contain water as a vehicle but do not contain alcohol. They are mainly used as vehicles e.g. chloroform water.

(b) Concentrated aromatic waters

Concentrated aromatic waters contain alcohol as a solvent for the volatile ingredients e.g. camphor water, concentrated peppermint water, concentrated caraway water, concentrated cinnamon water etc.

PREPARATION OF AROMATIC WATERS

Aromatic waters are prepared by any of the following methods :
- (a) By dilution method
- (b) By solution method
- (c) By distillation method

(a) By dilution method

By this method the aromatic waters are prepared by diluting the concentrated water with 39 times its volume of water. Aromatic waters prepared in this manner contain a small proportion, usually about 1.5% v/v, of alcohol (90 per cent).

(b) By solution method

To prepare the aromatic water by solution method, shake the corresponding volatile oil with 500 times its volume of purified water. Repeat the shaking several times during a period of about 30 minutes. Allow the mixture to stand for 12 hours or overnight and filter, if necessary.

Alternatively the volatile oil may be triturated with a sufficient quantity of purified talc, kieselguhr or pulped filter paper, then gradually add 500 times its volume of purified water with continuous stirring, and filter.

(c) By distillation method

In this method distil the drug or volatile oil with sufficient quantity of purified water until the specified volume of distillate has been collected. Shake the distillate thoroughly, allow to stand for 12 hours, filter to remove any excess of oil.

Examples of aromatic waters include chloroform water, camphor water, concentrated peppermint water, anise water, dill water, rose water, cinnamon water etc.

Exercise No. 1

Object

Prepare and supply 50 ml Chloroform Water I.P. 1966.

I.P. formula

Chloroform	2.5 ml
Purified water, sufficient to produce	1000 ml

Procedure

Add chloroform to purified water. Shake frequently until chloroform dissolves in the purified water.

Storage

Store in a well-closed container.

Category

Pharmaceutical aid.

Dose

15 to 30 ml.

Uses

Chloroform water is used as a pharmaceutical aid. Since it has flavouring, sweetening and preservative properties so it is used as vehicle in certain preparations meant for internal use and as menstruum for extraction of drugs.

Explanation

In this preparation chloroform is required to be shaken vigorously to sub-divide the chloroform in small globules to increase the surface area of chloroform by which the rate of dissolution will increase because the solubility of a solute in a solvent is directly proportional to the surface area.

A distributing agent is not required because the product is only half-saturated with chloroform, and the latter dissolves upon shaking vigorously for a few minutes.

Since chloroform is volatile in nature therefore chloroform water is required to be stored in a well-closed container to prevent the volatilisation of chloroform.

Exercise No. 2

Object

Prepare and supply 50 ml Camphor Water I.P. 1966.

I.P. formula

Camphor	1 gm
Alcohol (90 per cent)	2 ml
Purified water to	1000 ml

Procedure

Dissolve the camphor in alcohol (90 per cent). Add the solution in successive portions to the purified water. Shake well after each addition. Afterwards shake occasionally until all the camphor is dissolved.

Storage

Store in a well-closed container.

Category

Pharmaceutical aid.

Dose

15 to 30 ml.

Uses

Camphor water is used as a vehicle for liquid preparation due to its flavouring properties. It is also used as a carminative.

Explanation

The solubility of camphor is only 1 : 700 in water but it is freely soluble in alcohol i.e. 1 part of alcohol. In camphor water, the strength of camphor is 1 : 1000 that is near to saturation. Since camphor is very soluble in alcohol, so water is prepared by dissolving the camphor in alcohol and then this solution is added in small quantities to water with vigorous shaking after each addition. The addition of alcoholic solution to water yields a finely divided precipitates of camphor which redissolves easily on shaking. The alcohol acts as a distributive agent.

Water should not be added to the alcoholic solution of camphor because in that case whole of the camphor will be precipitated out which will not redissolve easily on shaking.

Camphor is volatile in nature so camphor water should be stored in a well-closed container to prevent the volatilisation of camphor.

Exercise No. 3

Object

Prepare and supply 50 ml Dill Water Concentrated I.P. 1966.

I.P. formula

Dill oil	20 ml
Alcohol (90 per cent)	600 ml
Purified water, sufficient to produce	1000 ml

Procedure

Dissolve the dill oil in the alcohol (90 per cent). Add sufficient purified water in successive small quantities, with vigorous shaking after each addition, to produce 1000 ml. Add 50 gm purified talc, shake and set aside for a few hours, shake occasionally and filter.

Storage

Store in a well-closed container.

Category

Carminative, flavouring agent.

Dose

0.3 to 1.0 ml.

Uses

Dill water, concentrated, is used as carminative and flavouring agent. Due to this reason it is commonly used in gripe waters.

Explanation

Concentrated aromatic waters contain alcohol as solvent. The oil is not soluble in water but it is freely soluble in alcohol (90 per cent) i.e. in equal volumes of alcohol 90 per cent. So firstly the oil is dissolved in alcohol 90 per cent and then purified water is added. Upon addition of water, the non-aromatic terpenes present in the oil are precipitated. Therefore vigorous shaking during each addition of water is necessary to redissolve any of the aromatic portion of oil that is temporarily precipitated.

Purified talc or French chalk is used as an absorbent. The preparation is allowed to stand for a few hours to allow the finely divided globules of oil to coalesce and occasional shaking is done to facilitate the absorption of undissolved oil by the purified talc.

Many of the volatile oils possess aromatic odour and taste due to the presence of aromatic substances in it which constitute only a very small part of the oil whereas the remainder is non-aromatic. The aromatic part is much more soluble in alcohol than the non-aromatic part containing insoluble terpenes. When alcoholic solution of a volatile oil is added to water the non-aromatic portion gets precipitated which is removed with purified talc by filtration.

This preparation contains volatile oil so to prevent the volatilization of the volatile oil it should be stored in a well-closed container.

Exercise No. 4

Object

Prepare and supply 50 ml Peppermint Water Concentrated B.P. 1968.

B.P. formula

Peppermint oil	20 ml
Alcohol (90 per cent)	600 ml
Purified water, sufficient to produce	1000 ml

Procedure

Dissolve the peppermint oil in the alcohol (90 per cent). Add sufficient purified water in successive small quantities with vigorous shaking after each addition to produce 1000 ml. Add 50 gm purified talc, shake and set aside for a few hours, shake occasionally and filter.

Storage

Store in a well-closed container.

Category

Carminative and flavouring agent.

Dose

0.25 to 1 ml.

Explanation

Explanation is same as discussed in Exercise No. 3.

2
Solutions

Solutions are liquid preparations meant for internal or external use. They are prepared by dissolving ingredient(s) in a suitable solvent usually water. Sometimes alcohol or glycerine is added as preservative or to facilitate solution formation. The solute used is usually non-volatile. They are issued sterile or unsterilised depending on the purpose for which they are intended.

Simple solutions are prepared by dissolving the solute in a suitable solvent. The solvent may contain other ingredients which stabilize or solubalize the active ingredient. Strong iodine solution is the representative example of simple solution which is prepared in this way.

Solutions differ from mixtures that they are meant for internal and external use whereas mixtures are meant for internal use. Solutions can be stored for a longer time but mixtures are extemporaneously prepared which should be consumed within 2-3 days. If necessity arises then fresh mixture should be prepared.

The examples of solutions include amaranth solution, aromatic solution of ammonia, strong ammonium acetate solution, cetrimide solution, sodium chloride solution, cresol with soap solution, aqueous iodine solution, weak iodine solution etc.

Exercise No. 5

Object

Prepare and supply 500 ml Sodium Chloride Solution B.P.C. 1968.

Synonym

Normal saline.

B.P.C. formula

Sodium chloride	9 gm
Purified water to	1000 ml

Procedure

Dissolve sodium chloride in sufficient amount of purified water to produce 1000 ml and filter.

Storage

It should be stored in well-closed containers.

Note : If the solution is issued as sterile, it should be prepared under sterile conditions. After preparation and filtration it should be transferred to the final container, which is then closed and sterilized by autoclaving.

Category

Electrolyte replenisher.

Explanation

Sodium chloride solution (0.9% w/v) is also known as normal saline solution which is used to make the preparation isotonic with blood serum, that is, the solution has the same osmotic pressure as blood serum, and therefore readily diffuses through the walls of small arteries, veins, and capillaries without causing dialation or collapse. Similarly the blood corpuscles are unaffected. Sometimes sodium chloride solution is also used as irrigation fluid.

Exercise No. 6

Object

Prepare and supply 50 ml Aqueous Iodine Solution I.P. 1966.

Synonym

Lugol's solution.

I.P. formula

Iodine	50 gm
Potassium iodide	100 gm
Purified water, sufficient to produce	1000 ml

Procedure

Dissolve potassium iodide and iodine in 100 ml purified water. Then add sufficient purified water to produce the required volume.

Storage

Since iodine is volatile in nature and it will slowly volatilise, so to prevent the volatilisation of iodine this solution should be stored in a well closed, iodine resistant container.

Uses

It is a source of iodine. Iodine is an essential element of our body, its deficiency leads to hypothyroidism which ultimately leads to development of goiter. The minimum daily requirement of iodine for an adult is 100 μg.

This solution is often used in the treatment of thyrotoxicosis. Due to the presence of iodine it can also be used as an antiseptic solution.

Dose

0.3 to 1.0 ml.

Explanation

Iodine is practically insoluble in water as its solubility in water is 1 : 2950 but in the presence of potassium iodide it becomes soluble due to the formation of new compounds known as polyiodides e.g. $KI \cdot I_2$, $KI \cdot 2I_2$, $KI \cdot 3I_2$, $KI \cdot 4I_2$. The reactions of potassium iodide with iodine are given below :

$$KI + I_2 \rightleftharpoons KI \cdot I_2 = KI_3$$
$$KI + 2I_2 \rightleftharpoons KI \cdot 2I_2 = KI_5$$
$$KI + 3I_2 \rightleftharpoons KI \cdot 3I_2 = KI_7$$

Potassium iodide is added only to increase the solubility of iodine. In the beginning the potassium iodide and iodine are dissolved in a small amount of purified water because iodine dissolves more quickly in concentrated potassium iodide solution. The solution so obtained is then diluted by adding more of purified water to produce the required volume.

Exercise No. 7

Object

Prepare and supply 50 ml Strong Ammonium Acetate Solution I.P. 1966.

Synonym

Liquor Ammoni Acetatis Fortis.

It contains 57.5% w/v of ammonium acetate (limit ± 2.5%)

I.P. formula

Glacial acetic acid	453 gm
Ammonium bicarbonate	470 gm
Ammonia solution strong	100 ml or sufficient quantity
Purified water, sufficient to produce	1000 ml

Procedure

Mix the glacial acetic acid with about 350 ml of purified water. To this add ammonium bicarbonate in small quantities at a time with continuous stirring until whole of it is dissolved. Then add sufficient amount of ammonia solution (little at a time) until one drop of the resulting solution diluted with 10 drops of water, gives a full blue colour with 1 drop of bromothymol blue solution and a full yellow colour with one drop of thymol blue solution. Then add sufficient amount of purified water to produce the required volume.

Storage

It should be stored in a well closed, lead free glass container.

Category

Diaphoretic.

Dose

1 to 4 ml.

Uses

Strong solution of ammonium acetate is used as a diaphoretic. Diaphoretics are the preparations which are used to lower the raised body temperature by increasing the excretion of body fluids in the form of sweat and urine.

Explanation

In this preparation two alkaline substances i.e. ammonium bicarbonate and ammonia solution strong are used because it is not possible to prepare the solution by reacting glacial acetic acid with ammonium bicarbonate alone because at certain point the reaction between these two substances ceases and the desired product is not produced so ammonia solution strong is used to complete neutralization of the acid and to make the preparation alkaline having pH between 7.6 to 8.1. The reactions which occur in this preparation are described below :

$$NH_4HCO_3 + CH_3COOH \rightarrow CH_3COONH_4 + H_2O + CO_2$$
$$NH_4OH + CH_3COOH \rightarrow CH_3COONH_4 + H_2O$$

Glacial acetic acid contains not less than 99% w/w of $C_2H_4O_2$ whereas acetic acid contains 33.0% w/w of $C_2H_4O_2$. So glacial acetic acid cannot be replaced with acetic acid. Either of the two i.e. ammonium bicarbonate or ammonia solution strong cannot be used in excess amount because in the former case the acid is not completely neutralised, moreover excess of ammonium bicarbonate will settle at the bottom and in the second case, to neutralise 453 gm of glacial acetic acid about 1000 ml of ammonia solution strong is required which will increase the volume of the preparation. So ammonia solution is used along with ammonium bicarbonate just to neutralize the acid required in the preparation.

Glacial acetic acid, somewhat diluted with water, must be used to produce a solution of the desired strength.

The pH of this preparation is adjusted by using two indicators i.e. bromothymol blue and thymol blue because these two indicators produce different colours at different pH as given below :

Bromothymol blue gives :

Yellow at pH 6 → Green → Blue at pH 7.6

Thymol blue gives :

Yellow at pH 8.0 → Blue at pH 9.6

Bromothymol blue checks the lower limit i.e. pH 7.6 and thymol blue checks the upper limit i.e. pH 8.0. Blue and yellow colours are obtained only between pH 7.6 to 8.0. Hence the neutral point specified lies between pH 7.6 and 8.0.

Exercise No. 8

Object

Prepare and supply 50 ml Chloroxylenol Solution B.P.C. 1968.

Synonyms

Roxenol.

B.P.C. formula

Castor oil	63.0 gm
Chloroxylenol	50.0 gm
Potassium hydroxide	13.6 gm
Alcohol (95 per cent)	200.0 ml
Terpineol	100.0 ml
Oleic acid	7.5 ml
Purified water to	1000.0 ml

Procedure

Dissolve potassium hydroxide in 15 ml water. Separately make a solution of castor oil in 63 ml of alcohol. Mix the two solutions and allow to stand for one hour or until a small portion of the mixture remains clear when diluted with 19 times its volume of purified water, and then add the oleic acid. Mix the terpineol with a solution of the chloroxylenol in the remainder of alcohol, pour into the soap solution, and add sufficient water to produce the required volume.

Alcohol content

16 to 20% v/v of ethyl alcohol.

Content of chloroxylenol

4.5 to 5.5% w/v.

Uses

As a germicidal agent. Chlorinated phenols have become very popular during recent years as germicidal agents. This is because some of them are less toxic and more germicidal than phenol or cresol. In general, the higher the molecular weight of the chlorinated phenol, the less toxic and more germicidal it is. Chloroxylenol is a good example of these compounds and is sufficiently soluble in properly formulated solutions to form an efficient germicide. Volatile oils or volatile substances are commonly added to mask the odour of the phenolic substances and the solubility of the latter is increased by adding a neutral soap to the preparation.

Explanation

1. In the preparation of this solution alcohol 95 per cent may be replaced by industrial methylated spirit.
2. Alcoholic solution of castor oil forms caster oil soap with potassium hydroxide (potassium ricinoleate) at a faster rate. It helps in solubalizing chloroxylenol and further acts as emulsifying agent when the solution is diluted with water.
3. Oleic acid neutralizes the solution to give optimum pH for bactericidal action.
4. Chloroxylenol and terpineol are only slightly soluble in water but are readily soluble in alcohol (95 per cent). Chloroxylenol is readily soluble in terpineol. The final percentage of alcohol in this solution is 20% which is insufficient to hold both the ingredients in solution. Soap forms micelles and solubalizes terpineol and chloroxylenol. So a clear colloidal solution is obtained.

3

Spirits

Spirits, also known as essences, are the alcoholic or hydroalcoholic solutions of volatile substances. The volatile substances used may be in the form of solid, liquid or gas.

They are used internally as well as externally by inhalation for their medicinal value while a large number of them are used as flavouring agents. These may be used in the formulation of aromatic waters or other pharmaceuticals in which flavour is required.

Spirits should be stored in air-tight, light-resistant containers and in a cool place to prevent the evaporation and volatilisation of alcohol or the active ingredients.

METHODS OF PREPARATION OF SPIRITS

Spirits can be prepared by any of the following methods :
- (i) Simple solution
- (ii) Solution with maceration
- (iii) Chemical reaction
- (iv) Distillation

(i) Simple solution

It is a simple procedure in which the volatile substances are dissolved in alcohol. Sometimes filtration is required to obtain a sparkling clear liquid. Spirits prepared by this method include ether spirit, chloroform spirit, peppermint spirit etc.

(ii) Solution with maceration

In this method, leaves of the drug are macerated in purified water to extract water soluble constituents. The marc is pressed and expressed liquid is mixed with the extract. Then sufficient quantity of alcohol is added and the liquid is filtered. The product possesses green colour due to the presence of soluble chlorophyll. Official peppermint spirit is made by this process but peppermint spirit B.P.C. is prepared by dissolving peppermint oil in alcohol only.

(iii) Chemical reaction

No official spirits are prepared by this method.

(iv) Distillation

Aromatic spirit of ammonia I.P. 1966 is prepared by this method.

Exercise No. 9

Object

Prepare and supply 50 ml Chloroform Spirit I.P. 1966.

I.P. formula

Chloroform	50 ml
Alcohol (90 per cent) sufficient to produce	1000 ml

Procedure

Mix chloroform with a small quantity of alcohol, then add more of alcohol to produce the required volume.

Alcohol content

83 to 87% v/v.

Category

Pharmaceutical aid.

Dose

0.3 to 1 ml.

Storage

It should be stored in a well-closed glass container in a cool place to prevent the volatilisation of volatile ingredients.

Uses

Chloroform spirit is used as sweetening agent, carminative and preservative. It is one of the main ingredients of carminative mixtures.

Explanation

Inhalation of chloroform causes anaesthesia. When chloroform is exposed to air and light, oxidation take place but the presence of alcohol in chloroform spirit retards the oxidation.

Exercise No. 10

Object

Prepare and supply 50 ml Peppermint Spirit B.P.C. 1968.

Synonym

Essence of Peppermint.

B.P.C. formula

Peppermint oil	100 ml
Alcohol (90 per cent) to	1000 ml

Procedure

Dissolve peppermint oil in a small amount of alcohol. To this add more of alcohol to produce the final volume. If the solution is not clear to this add 50 gm purified talc and shake, set aside for sometime and then filter to get the clear liquid.

Alcohol content

78 to 82% v/v.

Storage

It should be stored in a well-closed container and in a cool place to prevent the volatilisation of volatile ingredients.

Dose

0.3 to 2 ml.

Uses

It is used as carminative and flavouring agent.

Explanation

Official peppermint spirit is prepared by solution with maceration process but peppermint spirit B.P.C. is prepared by solution method in which peppermint oil is dissolved in alcohol.

Peppermint oil is obtained by distillation from the fresh flowering tops of *Mentha piperita* family *Labiatae*.

4
Tinctures

Tinctures are alcoholic or hydroalcoholic solutions usually containing comparatively low concentration, the active principles of vegetable drugs. Certain alcoholic solutions of chemicals were previously known as tinctures e.g. tincture of iodine, but now they are called solutions e.g. weak iodine solution or strong iodine solution.

Tinctures differ from spirits that the tinctures contain low concentration of active principles of vegetable drugs whereas spirits contain volatile substances only.

The name tincture is applied to alcoholic products made from drugs when :

(i) the product contains 45% or more of alcohol, tincture of ipecacuanha is an exception;

(ii) 4 parts by volume or more of the product represent 1 part by weight of the drug. Strong tincture of ginger is an exception, 2 parts by volume represent 1 part of the drug.

Increasing use of pure drugs isolated from animals, plants or prepared by synthetic processes has reduced the use of plant or animal extracts but even then tinctures are still commonly used where comparatively low potency and large dosage are recommended. Since tinctures contain alcohol so they are very stable preparations and can be stored for a long time without degradation, decomposition as loss of potency.

Alcohol from 20 to 90 per cent is widely used as menstruum in the extraction of drugs because :

(i) The medicinally active ingredients of many drugs are soluble in alcohol.

(ii) Alcoholic preparations remain stable for a long period of time without degradation, decomposition or loss of potency.

(iii) Alcohol precipitates gums and albuminous matter, therefore alcoholic preparations may be filtered to obtain a clear liquid.

PREPARATION OF TINCTURES

Generally tinctures are prepared by the following extraction processes :

(i) Maceration

(ii) Percolation

(i) Maceration

(a) Maceration process for tinctures made from organised drugs

Maceration is the extraction process in which the solid drug is placed in contact with whole of the menstruum in a closed vessel for 2-7 days with occasional stirring. The liquid is strained and marc pressed, adding the expressed liquid to the strained liquid. The combined liquids are clarified by decantation or filtration. Final volume is not adjusted.

Organised drugs are those drugs which have well defined cell structure. All the plant tissues constitute the organised drugs.

Here the volume is not adjusted to obtain uniformity of strength of the finished product. If the volume will be adjusted then the product would vary in strength with the apparatus used for expression.

Tinctures prepared by this method include tincture of orange, tincture of capsicum, tincture of lemon,

(b) Maceration process for tincture made from unorganised drugs

Unorganised drugs are the plant exudates which include resins or oleo-gum resins. For the preparation of tinctures from these drugs the ordinary maceration process described above is used with certain modifications as given below :

(a) The time period of maceration is reduced in certain cases.

(b) The marc is not pressed.

(c) The product is adjusted to volume.

Preparations made by this process include compound tincture of benzoin, tincture of myrrh, tincture of tolu etc.

(ii) Percolation

Percolation, also known as simple percolation, is another method of extraction of active constituents from the drugs used in the preparation of tinctures and liquid extracts. In this process the suitably comminuted drug is moistened with a sufficient quantity of menstruum, which is then packed in a percolator. The drug is allowed to remain in contact with the menstruum for 24 hours, then more of menstruum is added from the top and percolation is started. The required volume is collected, marc is pressed and expressed liquid is added to the percolate. The required volume is produced by adding more of menstruum and the mixed liquid is clarified by decantation or by filtration.

Various steps involved in percolation process are as follows :

(i) Size reduction or comminution of the drug.

(ii) Imbibation.

(iii) Packing.

(iv) Maceration.

(v) Percolation.

Tinctures prepared by percolation process include tincture of belladonna, compound tincture of cardamom, strong tincture of ginger etc.

Storage

Tinctures should be stored in tightly-closed containers protected from light and in a cool place.

Note : Tinctures whose active principles alter with time (e.g. aconite tincture, belladonna tincture, hyoscyamus tincture) should be discarded after one year.

Exercise No. 11

Object

Prepare and supply Orange Tincture I.P. 1966 using 25 gm fresh orange peel.

I.P. formula

Fresh orange peel, in thin slices   250 gm
Alcohol (90 per cent)   1000 ml

Procedure

Take fresh orange peel and cut into thin slices. Weigh the required quantity of thin slices and macerate it with whole quantity of alcohol in a covered vessel. Allow to macerate for 7 days with occasional stirring. Strain the liquid, press the marc and mix the expressed liquid to the strained liquid. Clarify the combined liquids by filtration.

Alcohol contents

73 to 78% v/v.

Storage

Store in a well-closed container protected from light and in a cool place to prevent the volatilisation and deterioration of active constituents.

Dose

2 to 4 ml.

Uses

It is used as flavouring agent.

Explanation

1. Fresh orange peel is the fresh outer part of the pericarp of the ripe or nearly ripe fruit of *Citrus aurantium* family *Rutaceae*.
2. The inner white portion of the peel is excluded because it gives bitter taste to the preparation. Fresh orange peel is used for extraction because it contains more volatile oil than the dry peel.
3. Orange tincture is a permanent non-extemporaneous product and can be made in quantity when fresh peel is available.
4. The peel is thinly sliced to expose the oil glands embodied therein and to expose more surface area to the action of solvent.
5. The vessel is closed to prevent the volatilisation of volatile oils and alcohol.
6. To effect solution of the volatile oils alcohol 70 per cent or more is required. Fresh orange peel contains a large proportion of water which dilutes alcohol 90 per cent used to 73-78 per cent v/v.
7. During maceration process occasional stirring is necessary to displace the saturated layers of menstruum around the drug. This leads to more effective extraction.
8. Filtration is necessary to remove insoluble cell contents which are introduced due to pressing of marc.
9. Adjustment to volume is not made to keep uniformity in strength of the finished product.

Exercise No. 12

Object

Prepare and supply 50 ml Benzoin Tincture B.P.C. 1968.

Synonym

Simple tincture of benzoin.

B.P.C. formula

Benzoin crushed	100 gm
Alcohol (90 per cent) to	1000 ml

Procedure

Macerate the benzoin crushed in 800 ml of alcohol for one hour with frequent agitation, filter and pass sufficient alcohol through the filter to produce the required volume.

Alcohol content

81 to 85 per cent v/v.

Storage

It should be stored in a well-closed container and in a cool place to prevent the volatilisation of volatile ingredients.

Uses

It is an ingredient of inhalations used in the treatment of catarrh of the upper respiratory tract. For this purpose about 5 ml of the preparation is added to warm water and the vapours are inhaled. When mixed with glycerine and water, the tincture may be applied locally for cutaneous ulcers, bedsores, cracked nipples, and fissures of the lips and anus.

Explanation

1. Benzoin is a balsamic resin obtained from Styrax benzoin, known in commerce as Sumatra benzoin. It contains benzoic and cinnamic acid esters of the alcohol benzoresinol; free benzoic and cinnamic acids.
2. Crushed benzoin is used to expose a large surface area to the solvent action of the menstruum and thus ensure complete extraction of the constituents.
3. Alcohol 90 per cent is used to effect solution of the volatile oils and resin. The alcohol strength in the final preparation is reduced due to dissolved oil and resin, and not due to dilution with water.
4. In the beginning 80% of the menstruum is used because the oil and resin which pass into solution occupy a variable volume. This is adequately covered by adding remaining amount of menstruum to the preparation.
5. The liquid is filtered to separate the alcoholic layer from the gummy matter.
6. Sufficient menstruum is passed through the filter to wash any adherent alcoholic liquid from the gummy matter.

Exercise No. 13

Object

Prepare and supply 50 ml Strong Ginger Tincture I.P. 1966.

Synonym

Essence of Ginger.

I.P. formula

Ginger, in moderately coarse powder	500 gm
Alcohol (90 per cent), sufficient to produce	1000 ml

Procedure

It is prepared by percolation process. Moisten the drug with a portion of the menstruum and set aside for 4-6 hours. Pack the moistened drug in the percolator. Pour sufficient menstruum onto the drug so as to saturate the column of drug throughout its length and also form a layer above it. Set aside for 24 hours.

Commence the percolation and collect the percolate in a vessel. Continue percolation until 3/4 of volume of the finished product is obtained. Test the percolate for complete exhaustion of the drug. Press the marc and add the expressed liquid to the already collected percolate. The total volume should be about 80-90% of the final volume. Add more of menstruum to produce the required volume. Allow the liquid to stand to settle the suspended particles. Decant or clarify the liquid by filtration.

Alcohol content

80 to 88 per cent v/v.

Category Carminative.

Dose 0.3 to 0.6 ml.

Storage

It should be stored in air-tight containers to prevent the volatilisation of volatile constituents.

Uses It is used as carminative and flavouring agent.

Explanation

1. Ginger consists of the rhizome of *Zingiber officinale* family *Zingibracae*.
2. Ginger, in moderately coarse powder, is used to expose an adequately large surface to the solvent action of the menstruum.
3. The oleo-resins present in the drug are not soluble in water or dilute alcohol hence, a strong alcohol must be used to effect extraction.
4. Before packing the drug in the percolator, moistening is done to swell the drug otherwise if the swelling takes place in the percolator it will lead to tight packing of the drug and percolation would not take place.
5. After packing the moistened drug in the percolator, sufficient menstruum is poured and allowed to set aside for 24 hours so that during this period much of the soluble matter passes into solution.
6. The marc is pressed to recover as much as possible of the menstruum. This practically does not contain any medicinally active constituents. It is done just for reasons of economy.
7. Filtration is done to remove the cell debris expelled by expression of the marc.

Exercise No. 14

Object

Prepare and supply 50 ml Compound Cardamom Tincture I.P. 1966.

I.P. formula

Cardamom seeds in moderately course powder	14 gm
Caraway, in moderately coarse powder	14 gm
Cinnamon, in moderately coarse powder	28 gm
Amaranth	5 gm
Alcohol (45 per cent), sufficient to produce	1000 ml

Procedure

This tincture is prepared by percolation process. Mix the powders and moisten them with a sufficient quantity of alcohol. Collect about 900 ml of the extract. Separately dissolve amaranth in small amount of alcohol. To this add glycerine. Incorporate the solution so formed to the collected extract. Add more of alcohol to produce the required volume. Filter, if necessary.

Storage

It should be stored in a well-closed container.

Category

Carminative.

Dose

2 to 4 ml.

Uses

It is used as carminative and flavouring agent.

Explanation

1. As the preparation contains more than one ingredient for extraction therefore it is termed as compound tincture.
2. Cardamom seeds recently removed from the capsules should be used for powdering because it contains the required volatile constituents. Already removed or stored seeds will contain less amount of volatile ingredients.
3. Moderately coarse powders are used to expose an adequately large surface to the solvent action of the menstruum, moreover in case of non-reduction the menstruum will trickle down from spaces without penetrating the drug tissues.
4. Imbibation is done to swell the drug before packing in the percolator. If dry drug is packed there will be air entrapment through which the menstruum will flow and may disturb the packing of the drug in the percolator thus obstructing smooth percolation.
5. Moistened plug of cotton wool is placed over the perforated disc so as to prevent the falling of the drug particles in the tap of percolator thus blocking the tap. Moistening of cotton wool is done to prevent the fibres to fall in the tap.

6. Packing of the moistened drug should be uniform. It should neither be too tight nor loose. Tight packing will not allow the menstruum to pass freely which will lead to slow extraction rate. Similarly loose packing will allow the menstruum to pass through quickly resulting in incomplete contact with the drug, hence less dissolution of active constituents.

7. After packing the material in the percolator a piece of filter paper is placed over top layer of the packed material. On the filter paper a small quantity of washed sand is placed to prevent disturbance of the packed material.

8. After packing the column, sufficient menstruum is added to saturate the material and allowed to set aside for 24 hours so that during this period much of the soluble matter passes into solution.

9. Under no circumstances the column is allowed to become dry otherwise cracks will appear in the packed column resulting in inefficient percolation.

10. Glycerine prevents the precipitation of tannins and hence increases the stability of the product.

11. Amaranth is used as colouring agent.

12. Filtration is done to clarify the liquid.

5

Extracts

Extracts are concentrated preparations of vegetable or animal drugs obtained by extracting the active constituent of the respective drugs with suitable menstruum. They are prepared by maceration or percolation process (already described) by using suitable solvents such as water, alcohol or solvent ether. The liquid so obtained is evaporated either whole or part of it to evaporate the solvent. The residual concentrates or powders are adjusted to the prescribed standards.

FORMS OF EXTRACTS

Depending upon the consistency the extracts are made in three forms, i.e.

(a) Liquid extracts
(b) Soft extracts
(c) Dry extracts

(a) Liquid extracts

Liquid extracts are usually of such a strength that one part by volume of the preparation is equivalent to one part by weight of the crude drug. The examples of liquid extracts include liquid extract of liquorice, liquid extract of nux vomica, liquid extract of belladonna, liquid extract of hyoscyamus etc.

(b) Soft extracts

Soft extracts are prepared by evaporating the extractive until a soft mass is obtained. Soft extracts generally tend to harden during storage and form tough masses which are difficult to handle in dispensing.

(c) Dry extracts

Dry extracts are usually prepared by evaporating the extractive to dryness under reduced pressure. If the active principle is of a potent nature and permits of an assay then adjustment to a definite strength should be done by dilution with an inert powder. The examples of dry extracts include dry extract of belladonna, dry extract of nux vomica, dry extract of hyoscyamus etc.

Storage

Extracts should be stored in a well closed, light-resistant containers and in a cool place.

Exercise No. 15

Object

Prepare and supply Liquorice Liquid Extract I.P. 1966 by using 100 gm liquorice powder.

I.P. formula

Liquorice, unpeeled, in coarse powder	1000 gm
Chloroform water	a sufficient quantity
Alcohol (90 per cent)	a sufficient quantity

Procedure

Exhaust the liquorice with chloroform water by percolation. Boil the percolate for 5 minutes and set aside for not less than 12 hours. Decant the clear liquid and filter the remainder. Mix the two liquids and evaporate until the weight per ml of the liquid at 20°C is 1.198 gm. Allow the liquid to cool. When cold, add one fourth of its volume of alcohol (90 per cent). Set aside for not less than four weeks and filter.

Storage

It should be stored in a well-closed container and in a cool place.

Category

Mild expectorant.

Dose

2 to 4 ml.

Uses

Liquid extract of liquorice is used in cough lozenges, cough pastilles and cough mixtures. It is also used to mask the taste of nauseous medicines, especially the alkali iodides, ammonium chloride, quinine etc.

Explanation

1. Unpeeled drug is used because it is cheaper than the peeled drug and is equally suitable for the preparation of an extract.
2. Water easily penetrates most of the vegetable tissues hence only a low degree of comminution is necessary.
3. Though the constituents of liquorice are soluble in water but the extraction process continues for a number of days during which fermentation of fermentable sugars present in liquorice may take place. So to prevent fermentation, chloroform water is used as vehicle instead of water, which acts as a preservative. Chloroform is selected because it is volatile, and can be evaporated at a subsequent stage of preparation.
4. The percolate is boiled for 5 minutes to coagulate the albuminous matter. If not removed at this stage, it would be precipitated during the subsequent evaporation and its removal from viscous liquid would be more difficult. Moreover an appreciable portion of the viscous liquid would adhere to the coagulated matter and the yield of the product would be considerably reduced.
5. Evaporation of the mixed liquids is done to adjust the weight per ml or sp. gravity. This is done to standardize the product on the proportion of total solids. This is the only satisfactory method of standardization for the preparation.

6. Alcohol 90 per cent is used to preserve the product. Without the addition of alcohol the fermentation of the product would immediately take place which will make the product unstable. Fermentation cannot take place in aqueous preparations containing 20% or more of alcohol. Therefore sufficient quantity of alcohol (about 20%) is added to preserve the preparation.

7. After mixing alcohol, the preparation is set aside because the substances in the evaporated liquid are water-soluble but not necessarily soluble in weak alcohol, therefore some precipitation occurs due to change in the character of the solvent.

Exercise No. 16

Object

Prepare and supply Belladonna Liquid Extract B.P.C. 1968 by using 100 gm of drug.

B.P.C. formula

Belladonna root, in moderately coarse powder	1000 gm
Alcohol (80 per cent)	a sufficient quantity

Procedure

Exhaust the drug with alcohol by reserved percolation process. Reserve the first 400 ml of percolate, evaporate the subsequent percolate under reduced pressure to the consistency of a soft extract and dissolve it in the reserved portion. Determine the proportion of total alkaloids. To this add sufficient alcohol 80 per cent to produce the extract of required strength. Allow to stand for not less than 12 hours and filter, if necessary.

Alcohol content

48 to 60 per cent v/v of ethyl alcohol.

Storage

It should be stored in a well-closed container, in a cool place and protected from light.

Uses

The use of belladonna liquid tract is due to the presence of its principal alkaloids hyoscyamine and atropine. Therefore this preparation is used to decrease secretions of sweat, salivary and gastric glands. It acts as a powerful spasmolytic in intestinal colic. It is also used for the relief of spasm associated with biliary and renal colic.

Explanation

1. This preparation is prepared by reserved percolation process. The percolation process is already described which involves comminution, imbibation, packing, maceration and percolation.

   Reserved percolation process is a percolation process in which first portion (about 3/4th of final product) of the percolate which contains the maximum amount of active constituents is reserved and subsequent percolation is completed as usual until the drug is exhausted but the last part, about 1/4th of final volume is collected separately. The second dilute part is then evaporated to get a syrupy consistency which is then mixed with the reserved portion of the percolate and the final volume is adjusted by adding more of menstruum.

   Reserved percolation process is used for the preparation of liquid extracts as they are more concentrated preparations as compared to tinctures prepared by simple percolation process. Generally alcohol is used as menstruum for reserved percolation process and first portion of percolate which contains the bulk of dissolved active constituents is reserved and only the last portion which is dilute is subjected to evaporation, the concentrated product of which is mixed with the reserved part.

   Advantages

   (i) The reserved part of percolate which contains the maximum amount of dissolve principles is not subjected to heat treatment for evaporation, only the dilute portion of percolate is evaporated.

(ii) This process is economical as whole of the percolate is not evaporated.

2. Moderately coarse powder of the drug is used to expose large surface of the drug to the menstruum action.

3. The percolate is evaporated under reduced pressure so as to minimise conversion of hyoscyamine into atropine, a less potent substance.

4. Alcohol 80 per cent is used as menstruum because it is the best solvent for alkaloids.

5. The proportion of belladonna alkaloids (calculated as hyoscyamine) in the combined evaporated and reserved percolates should be adjusted to 10.75% w/v of alkaloid by dilution with more menstruum.

6. After producing the required strength with more of menstruum the preparation is allowed to stand for not less than 12 hours because some precipitation may occur slowly due to adjustment to volume with the menstruum.

Further, during evaporation, part of the soluble matter in the portion of the percolate so treated may have been rendered insoluble by changes caused by heating.

6

Creams

Creams are viscous semisolid ointment-like preparations but have lighter body than the ointments. They may be oil in water type (aqueous creams) or water in oil type (oily creams). Due to the presence of water soluble bases in oil in water type creams they can be easily removed from the skin and clothings. The aqueous creams have a tendency to bacterial and mold growth, therefore a preservative must be added. Even if a preservative has been incorporated care must be taken for complete cleanliness of the apparatus used in the manufacture of creams and containers used for packing the creams. If this precaution is not observed and a cream contaminated with micro-organisms is applied to the broken skin, it may produce infection in the patient.

Preparation of creams

To prevent any contamination with micro-organisms the apparatus used in the preparation of creams must be thoroughly cleaned with soap and water and rinsed with freshly boiled and cooled water and finally dried in the oven. All hygienic precautions should be taken throughout the preparation and final transfer into the containers.

Containers and storage

Creams should be supplied in well-closed containers, which should prevent evaporation and contamination. They should be stored in a cool place. The collapsible tubes made of metal or plastics are most suitable for packing the creams. Ointment jars can be used. Aluminium tubes are not suitable for packing creams which are preserved with an organic mercury compound.

Exercise No. 17

Object

Prepare and supply 50 gm Cetrimide Cream B.P.C. 1968.

B.P.C. formula

Liquid paraffin	500 gm
Purified water, freshly boiled and cooled	445 gm
Cetostearyl alcohol	50 gm
Cetrimide	5 gm

Procedure

Melt cetostearyl alcohol over gentle heat. To this add liquid paraffin and warm. Separately dissolve cetrimide in purified water and warm it to almost same temperature (about 60°C) as that of melted substances. Add the warmed aqueous liquid to the melted mixture and stir thoroughly until cold. Pack in suitable containers.

Storage

Store in a well-closed container and in a cool place.

Category

Bactericide.

Uses

It is used as an antiseptic cream for the treatment of wounds and burns; for the pre-operative cleansing of the skin and for the removal of scabs and crusts in skin diseases.

Explanation

Cetrimide is a quaternary ammonium compound. It is a relatively non-toxic antiseptic with detergent properties. It is quite effective against gram-positive micro-organisms but less effective against gram-negative micro-organisms. Aqueous solutions and creams containing 0.1 to 1.0% cetrimide are quite commonly used in hospitals for the treatment of wounds and burns.

Freshly boiled and cooled water is used to prevent the contamination by micro-organisms.

Hygienic precautions should be taken during preparation and filling of the cream in the containers.

Exercise No. 18

Object

Prepare and supply 50 gm Proflavine Cream B.P.C. 1968.

Synonyms

Flavine cream; Proflavine emulsion.

B.P.C. formula

Liquid paraffin	673 gm
Purified water, freshly boiled and cooled	250 gm
Wool fat	50 gm
Yellow bees wax	25 gm
Proflavine hemisulphate	1 gm
Chlorocresol	1 gm

Procedure

Melt together yellow bees wax and wool fat. Separately dissolve chlorocresol in 600 gm of liquid paraffin with the aid of gentle heat, add it to the melted substances and mix thoroughly. To this, add proflavine hemisulphate previously dissolved in water and warmed to almost same temperature as that of melted substances. Lastly add the remainder of the liquid paraffin. Stir gently and thoroughly until cold.

Storage

Store in a well-closed container and in a cool place.

Uses

It is used as an antiseptic cream.

Explanation

1. Wool fat and yellow bees wax are used as emulsifying agents in w/o type emulsions. Wool fat is also known as anhydrous lanolin. It is practically insoluble in water but can absorb about 50% of its weight of water. Therefore it is used to absorb water in this preparation because the quantity of water present in the preparation is quite large. Bees wax also acts as a stiffening agent.
2. Liquid paraffin is used as a base and emollient.
3. Wool fat and bees wax are to be melted over low heat because overheating leads to decomposition of the substances.
4. Freshly boiled and cooled water is to be used to prevent microbial contamination and all hygienic precautions should be taken during preparation and filling of the cream in the containers. Proflavine hemisulphate is also known as neutral proflavine sulphate, proflavine and proflavine hemisulphate. It acts as a slow-acting antiseptic which is effective against many gram-positive and gram-negative bacteria. In concentrations of 0.1 to 1 per cent or aqueous solution it is used in the treatment of wounds or burns.

7
Cosmetic Preparations

From time immemorial, people have used cosmetics to enhance their personal appeal by using different kinds of preparations. The cosmetics which are widely used now a days include tooth pastes, tooth powders, mouth washes, shampoos, nail polishes and polish removers, face powders, cold creams, vanishing creams and talcum powder, etc.

According to Drug and Cosmetics Act, the cosmetics are defined as the articles which are intended to be rubbed, poured, sprinkled, sprayed, introduced in, or otherwise applied to any part of the human body for cleansing, protecting, beautifying, promoting attractiveness or altering appearance.

A cosmetic only cleans, beautifies, alters the appearance, adds fragrance or stops the development of bad odour. It changes, increases or decreases the colour but it does not have any medicinal effect on the body. Thus ordinary toothpastes and toothpowders are cosmetics since they are used to clean the teeth and impart a pleasant feeling to the breath. But if such dentifrices include drugs such as antibiotics, fluorides, ammoniated materials and other substances which bring changes in the oral cavity then these preparations can be called drugs although they may not cease to be cosmetics.

Soap is used by almost everyone and is considered more of a bodily necessity than a cosmetic but toilet and bath soaps are specifically excluded from cosmetics. Similarly preparations such as room deodorants, etc., are not cosmetics but if the same deodorant is applied on the body it is termed as cosmetic. The devices or toilet articles used in applying the cosmetics such as tweezers, razor blades and combs should not be included in cosmetics.

Most cosmetics are safe for use by most people but adverse reactions occur in many cosmetics such as deodorants/antiperspirants, hair removers, hair sprays, eye creams, hair colour/dye lighteners, facial skin creams/cleansers and nail polishes.

The cosmetics are mostly used by women and they are more concerned about the physical characteristics like texture, consistency, colour, odour, packaging and general appearance of cosmetics than chemical characteristics.

Exercise No. 19

Object

Prepare and supply 50 gm Tooth Powder.

Formula

Precipitated calcium carbonate	92.0 gm
Hard soap, powdered	50.0 gm
Saccharin	2.0 gm
Peppermint oil	4.0 ml
Cinnamon oil	2.0 ml

Procedure

Pass the solid substances through a fine sieve and mix them in the ascending order of their weights. To the mixed powders add the flavouring agents and mix thoroughly. Again pass through the sieve to remove lumps, if formed.

Storage

Store in a well-closed container.

Uses

This preparation is used as a tooth powder.

Explanation

1. Precipitated calcium carbonate is used as abrasive. Abrasives are the substances which are used to remove debris and residual stains from the teeth and for polishing the tooth surface.
2. Powdered hard soap is used to enhance the action of abrasives by wetting the teeth, the food particles, if any, and to emulsify the mucous.
3. Saccharin is used as a sweetening agent.
4. Peppermint oil and cinnamon oil are used as flavouring agents.

Exercise No. 20

Object

Prepare and supply 50 ml Calamine Lotion I.P. 1966.

I.P. formula

Calamine	150 gm
Zinc oxide	50 gm
Bentonite	30 gm
Sodium citrate	5 gm
Liquefied phenol	5 ml
Glycerin	50 ml
Rose water of commerce, sufficient to produce	1000 ml

Procedure

Mix the weighed amount of calamine, zinc oxide and bentonite in a mortar. Triturate it with a solution of sodium citrate in about 700 ml of rose water. Add the required quantity of liquefied phenol and glycerin; mix well. To this add more of vehicle to produce the required volume, mix thoroughly so as to get a uniform preparation.

Storage

Store in a well-closed container.

Uses

This lotion is used as an astringent and protective against sun burn. It acts as a soothening agent and gives relief from itching and pain during skin irritation. It is also used in ringworm infection and eczema.

Explanation

1. Calamine is basic zinc carbonate mixed with suitable amount of ferric oxide to impart pink colour. It is often prescribed by dermatologists to give flesh-like colour to lotion or creams.
2. Zinc oxide has mild astringent, protective and antiseptic action. It is widely used in dusting powders, lotions, and ointments meant for the treatment of skin diseases and infections such as eczema, ringworm, psoriasis (chronic skin disease in which red scaly patches develop) and pruritus (itching).
3. Bentonite is a native colloidal hydrated aluminium silicate. It is insoluble in water but swells up nearly seven times its bulk and forms a magma with desirable viscosity. Hence it is used as suspending agent for the dispersion of insoluble substances like calamine etc.
4. Sodium citrate is added to prevent the lotion from being too viscous. It acts as a buffer and maintains the pH appropriate for skin preparations.
5. Liquefied phenol acts as antipruritic because of its antiseptic properties and also because of its local anaesthetic action.
6. Glycerin acts as a hygroscopic thus keeps the skin moist and has soothening effect on the skin.

Exercise No. 21

Object

Prepare and supply 50 gm Cold Cream.

Formula

Liquid paraffin	20.0 gm
Hard paraffin	4.5 gm
Lanette wax	3.5 gm
Glycerin	4.5 gm
Water	17.5 gm
Propyl paraben	0.1 gm
Perfume—sufficient quantity	

Procedure

Melt the lanette wax, hard paraffin and liquid paraffin on water bath. Separately dissolve propyl paraben in water, add glycerin to it and heat this solution to almost same temperature (about 60°C) as that of melted bases. Mix both the solutions and stir continuously until cold and uniform product is obtained.

Storage

It should be stored in a well-closed container and in a cool place.

Uses

It is used as skin protective and skin smoothener.

Explanation

Lanette wax was originally a German patent and was widely used in dermatological preparations. It consists of a mixture of sodium cetostearyl sulphate (10 per cent) and cetyl and stearyl alcohols (90 per cent). For pharmaceutical purposes it is now largely replaced by emulsifying wax which is suitably prepared by mixing 90 gm of cetostearyl alcohol, 10 gm of sodium lauryl sulphate and 4 ml of water.

Lanette wax produces an oil in water emulsion. Propyl paraben acts as a preservative. Glycerin is used for water retaining and emollient properties. Liquid paraffin and hard paraffin act as base.

8

Capsules

Capsules are the solid unit dosage form of medicament in which drug(s) is enclosed in a practically tasteless, hard or soft soluble container or shell made up of a suitable form of gelatin. A preservative and colouring agent may be included in the formation of shells.

There are two types of capsules : (i) hard gelatin capsules which are generally used for filling the solid substances and (ii) soft gelatin or flexible capsules which are used for filling liquid and semi-solid preparations.

The hard gelatin capsules are made up of two cylindrical halves (i) longer and narrow half is called the base and (ii) shorter and wider half is called cap. The drug is filled into the base and cap is placed over it.

Hard gelatin capsules differ from soft gelatin capsules that they are hard in nature, used for filling solid substances and are manufactured in two stages where the shells are prepared at one stage and filling is done in the second stage. The hard gelatin capsules can be extemporaneously filled and cost of production is less. Whereas soft gelatin capsules are elastic in nature due to the presence of a plastisizer in the shell, are used for filling the liquid and semi-solid substances and preparation and filling is done in one stage only. Soft gelatin capsules cannot be prepared in the dispensary because it requires heavy machinery, hence the cost of production is more.

Exercise No. 22

Object

Prepare and supply 10 capsules of Compound Acetylsalicylic Acid.

Synonym

A.P.C. capsules.

Formula

Acetylsalicylic acid	300 mg
Paracetamol	150 mg
Caffeine	50 mg

Procedure

Powder a slight excess of the ingredients, if already not in powder form. Weigh the calculated quantities of each ingredient. Mix them in the ascending order of their weights.

Place the mixed powders on glazed tile or glazed paper in a layer about one-third of the height of the capsule in thickness. Remove the cap from the shell. Repeatedly press the inverted base of the capsule on the powder until the capsule is filled with the desired weight of the powder. Replace the cap over the base. Check the weight by keeping an empty shell in the other pan of the balance as a tare. Fill the required number of capsules. After filling, a small amount of the powder sticks to the sides of the capsule, if not removed produces bitterness and deliquescence, thereby whole aim of filling the drug into capsules is lost. Moreover the whole process involves much handling of the capsules which leaves fingerprints on the filled capsules. Therefore it is necessary to clean the capsules after filling. The most suitable method is to roll the filled capsules in dry towel, very lightly sprinkled with liquid paraffin. By this method sticking materials will be removed and it will also impart shine to the capsules.

Transfer the capsules in capsule vials, label and dispense.

Storage

Store in a well-closed container and in a cool place with controlled humidity. At higher temperatures the moisture is lost and the capsules become brittle and tend to crack. In a humid atmosphere the capsules absorb moisture and loose shape.

Dose

1 to 2 capsules.

Explanation

1. Acetylsalicylic acid is also known as aspirin. It is used as analgesic antipyretic, antirheumatic. Aspirin should not be given to children under one year of age except under medical supervision.
2. Paracetamol acts as an analgesic and antipyretic.
3. Caffeine is mainly obtained from coffee, it may also be prepared synthetically. It acts as C.N.S. stimulant. In some way it potentiates the actions of other ingredients.

Exercise No. 23

Object

Prepare and supply 10 capsules each containing 200 mg of Ferrous Succinate.

Procedure

Place the weighed amount of ferrous succinate on glazed tile or glazed paper in a layer about one-third of the height of the capsule in thickness. Remove the cap from the shell. Repeatedly press the inverted base of the capsule on the powder until the capsule is filled with the desired weight of the powder. Replace the cap over the base. Check the weight by keeping an empty shell in the other pan of the balance as a tare. Fill the required number of capsules. After filling clean and polish the capsules so as to remove the sticking powder outside the capsules and to impart shine to the capsules respectively.

Storage

These capsules should be stored in airtight containers protected from light.

Dose

Initial therapeutic dose 2-3 capsules (400-600 mg) daily and maintenance dose one capsule (200 mg) daily.

Explanation

1. Ferrous succinate is preferred over ferrous sulphate because it has less gastrointestinal side-effects.
2. To obtain maximum absorption, ferrous succinate capsules should be administered between meals.

9

Tablets

Tablets may be defined as the solid unit dosage form of medicament or medicaments with or without suitable diluents and prepared either by molding or by compression. They vary greatly in shape, size and weight which depends upon the amount of medicament and the mode of administration. Most commonly the tablets are disk shaped with convex surfaces but they are also available in special shapes like round, oval, oblong, cylindrical, square, triangular etc. They vary greatly in weight. The tablets for oral administration may weigh from 0.2 to 0.8 gm including the diluents but the tablets meant for administration other than oral route may be lighter or heavier.

Tablets are the most widely used solid dosage form of medicament because they offer a number of advantages to the patient, prescriber, manufacturer and the manufacturing pharmacist. Because of these advantages their popularity is continuously increasing day by day.

There are two types of tablets : (a) molded tablets which are prepared by molding the powders in a mold and (b) compressed tablets which are prepared with the help of tablet-making machine by applying pressure on the granules/powders.

There are three methods by which compressed tablets can be prepared :

1. Direct compression
2. Dry granulation
3. Wet granulation

Here only wet granulation will be described.

Wet granulation

Wet granulation is also known as moist granulation. During wet granulation the medicament or mixture of medicaments are mixed with diluent, if required. The mixed materials are moistened with a suitable liquid excipient until a coherent mass is obtained. The moistened material is passed through sieve No. 6 to 20 and the granules so formed are dried in an oven at a temperature not exceeding 60°C. The dried granules are again passed through a proper sieve to obtain the granules of required size. The granules are then mixed with other excipients like the second portion of disintegrants, lubricants and flavouring agents etc. The blended granules are thus ready for compression

Exercise No. 24

Object

Prepare granules for 100 tablets of Compound Sodium Bicarbonate I.P. 1966 and compress 50 tablets.

Synonym

Sodamint tablets.

I.P. formula

Each tablet contains :
Sodium bicarbonate	0.320 gm
Mentha oil	0.004 ml

Procedure

Prepare the granules of sodium bicarbonate by moist granulation. To the dried granules add the mentha oil previously dissolved in small quantity of alcohol, mix thoroughly and compress to obtain the tablets.

Storage

Preserve these tablets in a well-closed container and store in a cool place.

Dose

2 to 6 tablets.

Uses

It is used as an antacid. Compound sodium bicarbonate tablets should be allowed to dissolve slowly in the mouth.

Explanation

1. In the preparation of tablets the fine powders are not used but they are prepared in the form of granules which are then compressed. The granules so prepared have certain advantages over fine powders that :
    (i) The granules flow evenly through the hopper resulting in tablets of uniform weight whereas the fine powders do not flow evenly through the hopper which produces tablets of varying weights.
    (ii) The drugs are uniformly mixed and bound together in the form of granules thereby the mixed drugs do not separate out whereas in a powder containing several ingredients the vibrations of the machine separates the materials, the heavy materials move downward thereby the resulting tablets may not be uniform in composition.
    (iii) The very fine powders have a tendency to blow out of the die and stick to the sides of the punches. Granules being heavier do not have this difficulty.
    Proper size of the granules must be prepared. No. 12 to No. 20 mesh size granules are considered most suitable. It is not necessary that the whole material must be in granules, usually a small proportion 10 to 20% of fine powder must also be present which produces smoother tablets. Large size granules are not preferred because they may not feed into the dies as evenly or compress well as granules of proper size.
2. Since the quantity of sodium bicarbonate prescribed is sufficient therefore there is no need of adding any diluent.

3. As these tablets are required to be dissolved slowly in the mouth so a strong binding agent is to be added.

4. To prepare the granules a granulating agent is to be used. For this purpose 20% w/v acacia solution can be used which will serve both the purposes i.e. act as granulating agent as well as binding agent.

5. The quantity of mentha oil is very small which is not possible to be sprayed over the granules therefore it is first dissolved in alcohol 90% and then sprayed over the dried granules just before compression. It must not be added during granulation because in that case the oil will evaporate during drying the granules.

Exercise No. 25

Object

Prepare granules for 100 tablets of Calcium Lactate I.P. 1966 and compress 50 tablets each containing 300 mg of Calcium Lactate.

Procedure

Mix the weighed amount of calcium lactate with half the calculated quantity of starch. To this add sufficient quantity of 10% starch mucilage which will act as granulating agent and binding agent. Mix thoroughly so as to get wet coherent mass. Pass this wet mass through a sieve No. 10 to prepare the granules. Dry the granules in an oven at a temperature not exceeding 60°C. Pass the dried granules again through sieve No. 10 superimposed on sieve No. 20 to get the granules of proper size. Mix the granules so obtained with the second portion of disintegrating agent, lubricants and flavouring agents. The blended granules are thus ready for compression.

Storage

It should be stored in a well-closed container.

Dose

1 to 5 gm.

Uses

It is used in the treatment of calcium deficiency.

Explanation

1. The explanation for the preparation of granules is the same as described under Exercise No. 24.
2. As the quantity of calcium lactate is sufficient to be compressed therefore there is no need to add any diluent.
3. Calcium lactate is insoluble in water therefore a disintegrating agent is required to be added.
4. A granulating agent is used to prepare the granules. For this purpose 10% starch mucilage is used which acts as granulating agent and binding agent.
5. Disintegrating agent i.e. starch 5% is added in two stages one before granulation and the other after the granulation i.e. before compression. The second portion added helps in breaking the tablet in smaller particles whereas the first portion of disintegrating agent added before granulation helps in breaking the granules into still smaller particles.
6. Two sieves i.e. sieve No. 10 superimposed on sieve No. 20 are used to get the granules of proper size having sufficient amount of fine powder in it for easy and uniform compression of granules into tablets. The granules passed through sieve No. 10 but retained over sieve No. 20 are used for compression. The excess of fine powder which passes through sieve No. 20 is rejected.

10

Preparations Involving Sterilisation (Parenteral Preparations)

Parenteral preparations or injectables are the sterile solutions or suspensions of drugs in aqueous or oily vehicles meant for introduction into the body by means of an injection under or through one or more layers of the skin or mucous membrane. Since they are introduced into internal body compartments they must be sterile and free from all types of living micro-organisms and microbial products such as toxins, pyrogens etc. and should be free from particles like dust, fibres etc. They should be isotonic with body fluids. An utmost care must be taken in the preparation of injectables to avoid all types of physical, chemical or microbial contaminations.

Advantages

1. Parenteral route of administration is used when a rapid onset of action of the drug is required, hence this route is used in emergency cases.
2. This route is preferred when the drugs are inactivated in the G.I.T. or drugs are not well absorbed after oral administration.
3. This is the most suitable route of administration of drugs in treating patients who are non-cooperative, unconscious or are otherwise unable to take the medicine orally.
4. Prolonged action of a drug can be successfully produced by this route.
5. Solutions in volumes from fraction of a millilitre to 4 litres can be introduced by parenteral route.

Disadvantages

1. This mode of treatment is more expensive because it requires a technical and trained person for administration.
2. Sterilization is of utmost importance.
3. The administration of a drug through wrong route of injection may prove fatal.
4. Daily or frequent administration of injections may pose difficulties to the patient.

Exercise No. 26

Object

Prepare and supply 5 ampoules of 10 ml each of Dextrose Injection I.P. 1996.

I.P. formula

Dextrose	50 gm
Water for injection, sufficient to produce	1000 ml

Procedure

Dissolve dextrose in sufficient water for injection to produce 1000 ml. Filter the solution, if necessary. Distribute this solution in thoroughly cleaned and dried ampoules each containing 10 ml of dextrose solution. Care must be taken that during filling, the solution should not touch the sides of neck of ampoules; seal the ampoules and sterilise by moist heat sterilisation (autoclaving).

Storage

It should be stored in a cool place at a temperature not exceeding 25°C.

Dose

According to the need of the patient usually 5% w/v solution is administered but it can be introduced in concentrations of 10% and 20%.

Uses

It is used as nutrient replenisher thus act as readily available source of energy to the body. It is used to increase the volume of the circulating blood in shock and to counteract dehydration due to vomiting and diarrhoea. It is also given along with sodium chloride when desired to replace excessive salt loss due to vomiting.

Explanation

1. Since dextrose injection is to be introduced in the body by parenteral route therefore water free from pyrogens i.e. water for injection is used for the preparation of dextrose solution.
2. Dextrose solution can be sterilized by autoclaving or by filtration through bacteria-proof filters.
3. During filling the ampoules, the dextrose solution should not touch the sides of the neck of the ampoules because during sealing the ampoules, charring of dextrose may take place leading to the formation of black particles which may fall in the contents thus making them unfit for consumption.
4. If the ampoules show any colour, or contain a precipitate or any suspended impurities, they must be rejected.
5. As dextrose injection is a single dose container so bacteriostatic agent must not be added.

Exercise No. 27

Object

Prepare and supply 5 ampoules of 5 ml each of Sodium Chloride Injection I.P. 1966.

Synonym

Normal saline solution for injection.

I.P. formula

Sodium chloride	9 gm
Water for injection, sufficient to produce	1000 ml

Procedure

Dissolve sodium chloride in sufficient amount of water for injection to produce the required volume. Filter the solution, if necessary. Distribute this solution in required number of thoroughly cleaned and dried ampoules, seal them and sterilize in an autoclave as early as possible.

Storage

This injection on storage may lead to separation of small particles from the glass container. A solution containing such particles may not be used.

Uses

It is used as electrolyte replenisher. It is given intravenously along with dextrose injection to those patients who are unable to take fluids by mouth.

Sodium chloride injection is often given parenterally in the treatment of poisoning by mercurial salts, phenol and other substances eliminated by the kidneys, except where there is pulmonary oedema.

Explanation

1. 0.9% w/v solution of sodium chloride is known as normal saline solution.
2. Sodium chloride solution can be sterilised by autoclaving or by filtration through bacteria-proof filters.
3. Sodium chloride injections have a tendency that on keeping, separation of small particles from glass containers may take place. Solutions containing such particles must not be used.

11
Ophthalmic Preparations

These are the preparations which are to be instilled into the eye in the space between the eyelids and the eyeballs. They may also be injected into various regions of the eye. Though they are not parenterals by definition but have many similar and often identical characteristics.

Ophthalmic preparations must be sterile and are prepared under the same conditions and by the same methods as other parenteral preparations. Solutions used during surgery must be sterile and should not contain any preservative. They should be supplied in single-use containers and any solution remaining at the end of the operation must be discarded.

Since the capacity of the eye to retain liquid and ointment preparations is limited so they are generally administered in small volumes. Various ophthalmic preparations include :

1. Eye drops
2. Eye lotions
3. Eye suspensions
4. Contact lens solutions
5. Eye ointments
6. Ophthalmic inserts

Here only eye drops and eye lotions will be discussed.

Eye drops

Eye drops are sterile aqueous or oily solutions or suspensions for instillation into the eye. They are usually applied into the space between the eyeball and eyelids or onto the corneal surface. The main requirement of the eye drops is that they should be sterile, usually isotonic, buffered and free from foreign particles to avoid irritation to the eye. They usually contain substances having antiseptic, anti-inflammatory, mydriatic or miotic properties or substances used for diagnostic purposes.

Eye drops should be supplied in glass or suitable plastic containers with a screw cap fitted with a rubber teat and glass dropper for easy application of the drops or the containers may be fitted with a narrow nozzle from which the drops can be directly instilled into the eye.

Eye lotions

Eye lotions or eye washes are sterile aqueous solutions used for irrigating the eye. Sodium chloride eye lotion is used to remove foreign substances from the eye. They are usually applied with a clean eye-bath or sterile fabric dressing and a large volume of solution is allowed to flow quickly over the eye.

Eye lotions are usually supplied in concentrated form and are required to be diluted with an equal volume of warm water immediately before use. They should be freshly prepared and should not be stored for more than 2-3 days as they may be contaminated with micro-organisms on prolonged storage. Eye lotions should be isotonic and free from foreign particles to avoid irritation to the eye. The drugs used for preparing eye lotions include sodium chloride, sodium bicarbonate, boric acid, borax or zinc sulphate.

Exercise No. 28

Object

Prepare and supply 10 ml of 10 per cent Sulphacetamide Eye Drops B.P.C. 1968.

B.P.C. formula

Sulphacetamide sodium	10 gm
Sodium metabisulphite	0.1 gm
Phenylmercuric nitrate	0.002 gm
Purified water	100 ml

Procedure

Under aseptic conditions, dissolve sulphacetamide sodium in small amount of purified water. To this dissolve sodium metabisulphite and phenyl mercuric nitrate. Add more of purified water to produce the required volume.

Sterilize the solution by passing through a bacteria-proof filter. Transfer the solution to sterile container, which is then closed and sealed so as to exclude micro-organisms.

Storage

It should be protected from light i.e. the preparation should be supplied in light-resistant amber coloured bottle.

Uses

It is mainly used for local application in infections and injuries of the conjunctiva.

Explanation

1. The whole process from preparing the solution to sealing the container should be carried out under aseptic conditions.
2. Sulphacetamide eye drops in concentrations of 10%, 20% and 30% w/v may be used.
3. It is also used in the form of an eye ointment.
4. Sulphacetamide solution cannot be sterilized by autoclaving because on heating, hydrolysis of sulphacetamide takes place with the formation of sulphanilamide, which may be deposited as crystals, specially in concentrated solutions and under cold storage conditions.
5. When solution of sulphacetamide sodium comes in contact with light, discoloration of solution takes place which can be retarded by the addition of sodium metabisulphite and protection from light.
6. Phenylmercuric nitrate acts as a preservative.

Exercise No. 29

Object

Prepare and supply 200 ml Sodium Bicarbonate Eye Lotion B.P.C. 1968.

B.P.C. formula

Sodium bicarbonate	35 gm
Purified water	1000 ml

Procedure

Under aseptic conditions, dissolve sodium bicarbonate in purified water in a thoroughly cleaned container. Sterilise the solution by passing through bacteria-proof filter, transfer the solution to the final sterile container, which is closed immediately so as to exclude micro-organisms.

Storage

It should be stored in a cool place.

Uses

It is used as an eye lotion and as a first-aid treatment for irrigating burns.

Explanation

1. The whole process from preparing the solution to sealing the container should be carried out under aseptic conditions.
2. Sodium bicarbonate eye lotion should be used undiluted.
3. When a solution of sodium bicarbonate is sterilised by heating in an autoclave, carbon dioxide is first passed through the solution in the final container which is then hermetically sealed and not opened until at least two hours after the solution has cooled to room temperature.

12
Preparations Involving Aseptic Techniques

Aseptic technique by itself is not a process of sterilization but is a procedure that does not allow the bacteria to introduce into the preparation from possible sources of contamination such as ingredients, solvents, mixing equipment, final containers, the working area and operator's hands and other contact parts.

Whenever any work is to be done aseptically, it must be performed in an area free from micro-organisms known as aseptic area or in a room called aseptic room and the process so followed is called aseptic technique. The aseptic room has double door entry which are fitted with U.V. lamps. These lamps are also fitted above the working place. The operator should scrub his hands thoroughly with alcohol etc. and wear sterilized gloves, headgear, mask and clothings. All the apparatus and equipment required to be used in the process must be sterilized in advance.

For small scale work, where aseptic rooms are not available i.e. for extemporaneous preparations, aseptic chamber is used. Now a days, laminar air flow equipment is used for aseptic work which produces a very clean, dust and micro-organism free area. Various types of laminar air flow devices in the form of rooms, cabinets or benches are available.

The aim of aseptic technique is to prevent contamination of materials, instruments, utensils, glass apparatus etc., during handling. The utensils and glass apparatus should be thoroughly washed with soap and water to remove dirt and grease, then they are sterilized. After sterilization they should be removed from the oven/autoclave and stored immediately under aseptic conditions for future use.

Likely sources of contamination include air, breath, hair, clothes, hands and working surfaces. This contamination may be minimised :

(i) By introducing sterilized air under pressure into the working area.

(ii) By wearing sterilized gowns, face masks and gloves.

(iii) Hair should be covered with a sterilized cap and long hair should be tied at the back and covered.

(iv) The skin should be thoroughly washed with soap and water and then any suitable antiseptic solution applied thereon.

(v) Before starting the aseptic work the working surfaces of table or bench should be scrubbed with a swab of disinfectant.

(vi) Whenever strict aseptic conditions are required, a number of bunsen burners may be lit around the working place. Preferably a gas lighter should be used for lighting the burners and match stick or paper ignited from another burner should never be used because it will scatter particles into the air.

Exercise No. 30

Object

Prepare and supply 10 gm Chloramphenicol Eye Ointment B.P.C. 1968.

B.P.C. formula

Chloramphenicol	1 gm
Eye ointment base, sufficient to produce	100 gm

Preparation

The apparatus used in the preparation of eye ointment must be thoroughly cleaned and sterilized and the whole operation of preparation must be carried out under aseptic conditions. A formula for the preparation of eye ointment base is given below :

Yellow soft paraffin	800 gm
Liquid paraffin	100 gm
Wool fat	100 gm

Melt together the wool fat, yellow soft paraffin and liquid paraffin, filter while hot through a coarse filter paper in a heated funnel, sterilise by heating at a temperature of 160°C for one hour, and allow to cool, taking precautions to avoid contamination with micro-organisms.

Eye ointments are prepared by means of aseptic technique by using suitable method of preparation.

Powder the sterile chloramphenicol and thoroughly mix it with a small quantity of the melted sterile eye ointment base and then add the remainder of the sterile eye ointment base. Transfer the eye ointment to the final sterile container which is then closed immediately so as to exclude micro-organisms.

Storage

It should be protected from light and stored in a cool place.

Uses

It is an antibiotic which has a wide range of antimicrobial activity therefore used in the treatment of a wide variety of infections of the eye.

Explanation

1. For the preparation of eye ointment base, yellow soft paraffin is used instead of white soft paraffin because white soft paraffin is prepared by bleaching the yellow soft paraffin and bleaching agent may remain sticking to the white soft paraffin even after thorough washing which may lead to irritation to the eye.

2. For eye ointments intended to be used in tropical or subtropical climates, the proportions of paraffins may be adjusted according to the climatic conditions.

3. When the strength of the eye ointment is not specified, an eye ointment containing 1.0 per cent of chloramphenicol shall be supplied.

Exercise No. 31

Object

Prepare and supply 10 gm Chlortetracycline Eye Ointment B.P.C. 1968.

B.P.C. formula

Chlortetracycline hydrochloride	1 gm
Eye ointment base, sufficient to produce	100 gm

Procedure

The apparatus used in the preparation of eye ointment must be thoroughly cleaned and sterilized and the whole operation of preparation must be carried out under aseptic conditions.

The formula and method of preparation of eye ointment base is described under Exercise No. 30.

Finely powder the sterile medicament and thoroughly mix it with a small quantity of the melted sterile eye ointment base, then add the remainder of the sterile eye ointment base. Transfer the eye ointment to the final sterile container which is then closed immediately so as to exclude micro-organisms.

Storage

It should be protected from light and stored in a cool place.

Uses

It is an antibiotic which has a wide range of antimicrobial activity therefore used in the treatment of a wide variety of infections of the eye.

Explanation

When the strength of eye ointment is not specified, an eye ointment containing 1 per cent of chlortetracycline hydrochloride shall be supplied.

NOTES

NOTES

NOTES